WHY WOMEN EXPERIENCE MORE PAIN THAN MEN

and what

to do

about it

RUCSANDRA MITREA

Copyright 2024 by Rucsandra Mitrea

All rights reserved. No part of this book may be used or reproduced without the author's permission, except for brief quotations in articles and reviews and specific noncommercial uses permitted by copyright law.

Author photographs by The Likely Creatives
https://www.thelikelycreatives.com
Images copyright by Canva

First edition 2024

TABLE OF CONTENTS

INTRODUCTION — 5

YOU HOLD THE KEY! — 4

PART 1 - THE HIDDEN CAUSES OF PAIN — 7

THE PILLARS OF HEALTH ARE NOT ENOUGH — 8

WHAT IS GOING ON? — 9

THE DISCONNECTED STATE — 14

THE CONSEQUENCES — 18

PART 2 - RECLAIM YOUR BODY — 20

IT'S TIME! — 21

YOUR SUPERPOWER: AWARENESS — 23

PRACTICE GUIDE FOR YOUR BODY — 26

PRACTICE GUIDE FOR YOUR MIND — 38

PRACTICE GUIDE FOR YOUR EMOTIONS — 48

FINAL THOUGHTS — 56

INDESTRUCTIBLE CONFIDENCE — 57

WHAT'S NEXT? — 61

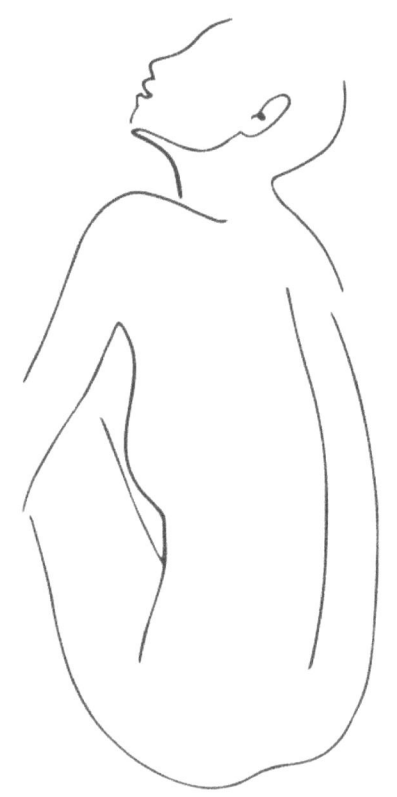

"Our own body is the best health system we have—if we know how to listen to it."

Dr. Christiane Northrup

ABOUT THE AUTHOR

Rucsandra Mitrea, a passionate and visionary teacher, guides women to access their power through understanding their bodies. With an impressive 30 years of experience, extensive research, and many certifications in various movement and healing modalities, Rucsandra has honed her expertise and developed a unique methodology for unlocking and harnessing a woman's connection with her body.

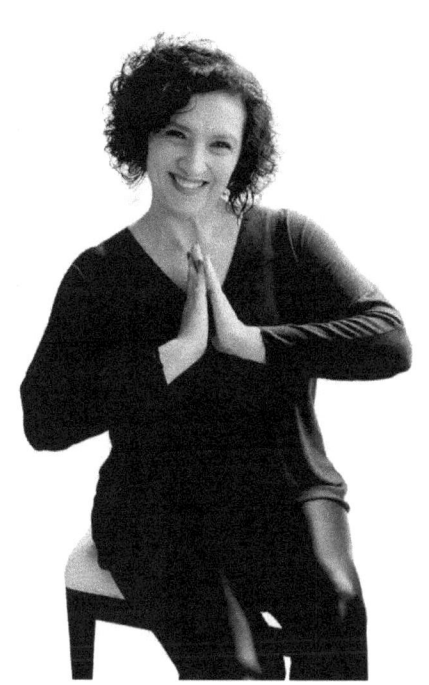

She is the author of "You Don't Have to Live in Pain: Five Strategies to Help Reduce Your Chronic Pain Right Now" and a contributing author to "Holistic Wellness In The NewAge: A Comprehensive Guide To NewAge Healing Practices."

In Rucsandra's words, "When women develop their ability to listen to their bodies, they not only experience a sense of freedom and liberation physically, mentally, and emotionally, but they also undergo a profound transformation in their self-awareness and approach to life. Ultimately, this journey *helps them regain their health, confidence, and power.*"

INTRODUCTION

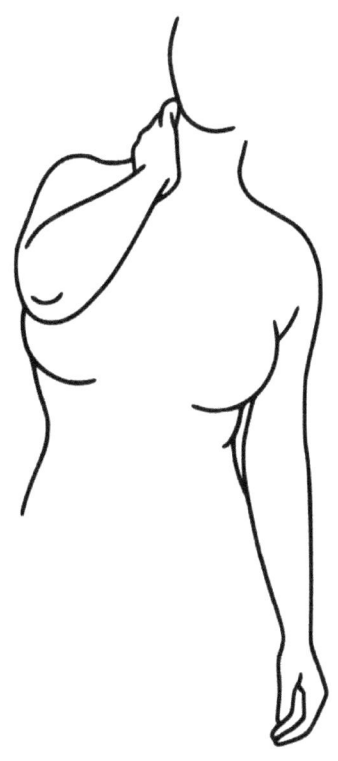

If you are currently reading this book, you have likely gone through physical pain in your life. I can relate, as I've lived with pain for more than half of my life. Multiple ankle sprains in my youth led to chronic inflammation in my ankles and knees, restricting movement and causing pain in my hips and lower back. In my early thirties, a herniated disc in my lumbar spine led to persistent low back and hip pain.

During my quest for physical healing, I dedicated a significant amount of time to researching and studying various healing modalities and movement therapies. Although I did notice some improvements in my body over time, I eventually realized that there was something more fundamental than any healing technique or method. It was only when I shifted my focus towards this discovery that I was ultimately able to completely reorganize and heal the injured tissues and joints and eliminate all discomfort and pain.

I felt like I had uncovered a remarkable secret that completely transformed my relationship with my body. This discovery enabled me to establish trust and confidence in my body's ability to heal itself. Later, when I was in my forties, this knowledge helped me to heal once again without having to undergo any invasive procedures or surgeries that the specialist recommended.

This secret is, in fact,

an innate superpower that all women possess

but are generally unaware of.

As a result, they experience increasing limitations, discomfort, and pain for years, even decades.

If you are struggling with discomfort or pain or with the so-called "age-related" limitations, it is not your fault for not knowing what I am about to reveal to you.

Injuries and the physical aging process are not the problem.

The problem lies in our education systems, upbringing, and culture.

This is the most significant missing information about women, our bodies, and our health.

Our doctors don't discuss it; some physicians don't even know its paramount importance in healing and aging in a strong, capable, and vital body—as a woman.

We were not taught about it in school, we didn't hear conversations about it in our family, we did not see it in the news, nor did we read about it in books as we grew up.

YOU HOLD THE KEY!

I want you to know that you can feel better no matter what is happening in your body or how unattainable a state of physical ease and joyful vitality may seem. In fact, you can feel a LOT BETTER than you have in years or even decades.

You can rise above your current situation and transform your body and life, regardless of age or past experiences.

This book doesn't present and explain concepts solely at an intellectual level. It is a manual—*an experiential guide*—with practical exercises to help you access and wield the power of the connection between your mind, body, and emotions.

I've written this book in two parts.

The first part explores the two hidden causes of pain. Women tend to experience pain more frequently and with greater intensity than men, and the root of this issue dates back centuries. This section provides a foundation for understanding your superpower and why it is vital to acknowledge and restore it.

The second part explains how to begin trusting your body. It contains three practice guides: one for your body, one for your mind, and one for your emotions. The exercises are designed to help you understand the connection between your body, mind, and emotions, not only at an intellectual level but also *in your body*.

The time is NOW to activate your superpower and reclaim your body. I will show you how.

Are you ready to learn about a woman's secret key to health and vitality at any age?

Are you ready to let go of feelings of powerlessness and embrace a powerful relationship with your body?

Are you ready to harness your superpower?

Let's get started!

PART 1

The Hidden Causes of Pain

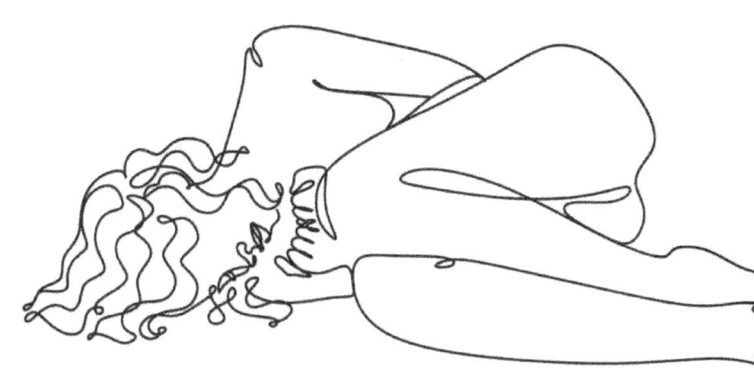

THE PILLARS OF HEALTH ARE NOT ENOUGH

Experts list some pillars of healthy aging: healthy nutrition, proper hydration, quality sleep, daily exercise and physical activity, relaxation, stress management, mental stimulation, social interaction, and meaningful relationships.

Women committed to staying healthy and active as they age are doing it all: they eat nutritious foods and limit sugar and other inflammatory substances, stay hydrated, sleep enough hours, exercise a few times a week, meditate, and spend time with friends and family.

However, statistics reveal an *unsettling reality*:

- 25% of Americans over the age of 55 have constant knee pain ([1](#))
- 20% of Canadians live with chronic pain ([2](#))
- 70% of American adults aged 50-80 experience symptoms of arthritis and joint pain ([3](#))

Over the past three decades of working with women, I have noticed that they tend to experience pain more frequently and with greater severity than men do.

Researching the statistics, I found that indeed:

- Women have more frequent, longer-lasting, and severe pain than men ([4])
- Chronic musculoskeletal pain is more common in females than males ([5])
- Females were consistently more likely than males to report pain or discomfort that prevents activities ([6])

To understand the root causes of this phenomenon, let's delve deeper.

My question is: if the pillars of health mentioned above hold the keys to healthy aging, why are so many women struggling with discomfort, pain, and increasing limitations?

And why is the percentage higher for women than for men?

WHAT IS GOING ON?

This widespread situation is occurring because women are not inherently taught how to understand and connect with their bodies to interpret their signals and messages correctly.

Many **women live in a state of disconnection** where their bodies, minds, and emotions are separate entities. This disconnection robs them of their well-being, health, and vitality; it robs them of the radiance they were born with *and profoundly alters their relationship with their body.*

The disconnection between mind, body, and emotions has been the default state for women for hundreds of years, not because this is a woman's natural state but because *women have been conditioned this way throughout centuries.*

A woman's mind, emotions, and body

are interconnected,

yet societal conditioning often leads

to them being experienced

as separate entities.

The roots of this conditioning are deeply ingrained in our past, stemming from two main paradigms: the separation between the mind and the body and the patriarchal rules and way of life. Let's explore them briefly.

1. THE SEPARATION BETWEEN THE MIND AND THE BODY

Since the 16th century, the Cartesian dual theory has defined our understanding of the world. French philosopher René Descartes (1596-1650) argued that the *body and the mind have different natures, are entirely different, and can exist independently*. Cartesianism involves oppositional pairs of concepts like mind/body, good/evil, and nature/culture rather than a more integrated way of understanding our bodies and our world.

The Cartesian dual theory has shaped our culture for the last six centuries and determined how we perceive and understand life. At the level of our society, it shaped our beliefs about health, disease, and healthcare systems.

Despite the many scientific advances in the last few decades that reveal the—unbreakable, irrevocable, and inalienable—connection between the mind and the body, it is not yet an essential part of our lives.

Although many women are familiar with the concept of the mind-body connection and its positive effects on their health and well-being, they still need to internalize it fully. In other words, they may understand it intellectually but have yet to experience it in their bodies before they can harness its power.

2. THE PATRIARCHAL RULES AND WAY OF LIFE

Centuries of patriarchal dominance have created and shaped systems of social relationships, values, norms, and behaviours that *infiltrated and still control every single aspect of a woman's life*. For centuries, women have been expected to mould their bodies, thoughts, beliefs, emotions, actions, and lives to fit the patriarchal rules and way of life.

The patriarchal conditioning has contorted, distorted, and imprisoned the consciousness of women, severing them from their natural understanding of the interconnectedness between their minds, bodies, and emotions, leaving them disconnected from themselves, without the means to access their innate wisdom and power.

Most women think, believe, act, work, exercise, and create their lives following masculine concepts and masculine practices that further disconnect them from their bodies, health, vitality, and radiance.

With both Cartesian and patriarchal determining factors, imbalance and disconnection are pervasive in all aspects of a woman's life:

- Her work and career
- Her money and finances
- Her leisure and pleasure
- Her spiritual practices
- Her relationships
- Her physical, mental, and emotional health

This book explains how, once and for all, you can transform your understanding of your body and return to your natural state, where mind, body, and emotions are intrinsically connected and inseparable.

First, we will explore the consequences of living in a disconnected state.

THE DISCONNECTED STATE

Living in a state of disconnection alters your relationship with your body. This leads to difficulties in accurately interpreting messages from your body, ultimately affecting your health and well-being.

I have created a list of ways the disconnected state may manifest in your body—notice which ones apply to you.

1. **You are only aware of your body when something hurts**, and so you are mainly noticing:

   - Sensations of pain and discomfort
   - Restrictions in ease of movement
   - Limitations in the range of movement
   - Loss of agility and balance
   - A combination of the above

This means that the counterbalance of noticing when you feel good, when your body is relaxed, or when an area of your body has significantly improved is not present in your awareness with the same level of clarity. *This further means that when something hurts, you focus mainly on the discomfort. You might not notice minor improvements or dismiss them as not good enough, making you feel more frustrated with your body and yourself.*

2. **You can't recognize your body's more subtle messages,** *which means you don't realize that many things that are supposed to get you positive results can adversely affect your body. For example, you may continue to run or go to the gym, even when your knees are inflamed and painful.*

3. **You may misinterpret your body's signals when it tells you to slow down or rest.** Instead, you might see it as a challenge to do even more, whether running longer, working out harder, or accomplishing more in general. *This can lead to pushing yourself too far, potentially resulting in repetitive injuries.*

4. **You may mistake your body's signals when it tells you to exercise regularly or go for walks.** Instead, you attribute your stiffness and soreness to aging and end up discouraged and frustrated.

5. **You may not be able to accurately distinguish between various sensations like soreness, ache, tenderness, and discomfort.** *As a result, you may end up labelling all of them as pain, causing you to think that you are in pain most of the time.*

6. **It's common to mistake the tension caused by emotional strain and stress with actual physical tightness.** *Therefore, attempting to stretch the tight parts of your body can lead to increased tension and more restriction over time rather than providing relief.*

7. **In daily life, you may not be mindful of your breathing**, which means you cannot use your breath in specific ways that effectively relax your body, calm your nervous system, and significantly diminish tension and discomfort. *Poor breathing habits can lead to increased stress and tension, which increase discomfort and pain in the long run.*

8. **You are not feeling much relief from discomfort and pain even after engaging in activities that are supposed to help**, such as working out, stretching, or following prescribed exercises by trainers or physiotherapists. *This means you may be investing a lot of time, resources, and effort without seeing any significant improvement.*

9. **You tend to accept that specific physical changes to your posture and lack of energy are consequences of aging**, even if you exercise regularly. For instance, you may notice that your upper back is rounded, your head is too far forward, or your lower back is arched, but you may feel helpless and believe that nothing can be done to fix them. *Consequently, you continue to exercise without paying attention to these issues, not knowing how to correct them, and hoping for the best.*

10. **Over years or decades of working out, it is possible to suffer from injuries, painful lower back conditions, damage to your neck or shoulders, severe arthritis to your knees or hips, and other related**

conditions. *This means that even though you may have worked hard to stay healthy and fit, your body may have suffered significant damage.*

11. **You are unaware of how different mental and emotional states affect the sensations and tension in your body**, which can lead you to believe that the discomfort or pain you may be feeling is solely related to your physical body. *As a result, you focus only on your body and try to fix something physically that has emotional causes. When the physical manifestations don't significantly improve, you may believe your body is at fault and failing you.*

And the list is far from over. These are just a few manifestations of the mind-body-emotions disconnect as they relate to how you connect with and understand your body.

THE CONSEQUENCES

The consequences of living in a disconnected, disembodied state are preventing you from moving and living with ease because they lock in patterns of restriction, limitation, and wear-and-tear in your body. They also don't allow you to correct the conditions leading to discomfort and pain. And they don't allow you to stave off the so-called age-related issues, even though you exercise regularly and do things meant to be good for your body.

You may be doing everything you can to help your body feel better, move better, and heal without considering your mental and emotional states and how they affect your body.

You may have exercised for years or decades, running, weightlifting, or doing Pilates or yoga, and you can lift an impressive amount of weight, perform complicated movements, or contort your body in complex poses. However, you're still hunched over and stiff and complain of back, neck, or hip pain. *Despite your dedication to fitness, your body may not be moving efficiently, causing discomfort or pain.*

And this is NOT health and vitality! It is the slow—and eventually painful—wear-and-tear and disintegration of your body year after year and decade after decade.

In my 30 years of helping women relieve discomfort and pain, I have observed firsthand how this disembodied state leads them to feel frustrated with their bodies and themselves, resentful, and disappointed.

Many women engage in physical activities that harm their joints, tissues, and overall health. They often push themselves beyond their limits, even when their bodies need rest and recovery. This pursuit of fitness can lead to severe pain, hip or knee replacements, or surgeries on the neck and lower back later in life.

Many women need to be more active but don't know where to start, are afraid of injuring themselves, are overwhelmed by the many available options, put everybody else's needs first, and don't make time for themselves.

A woman living in a disconnected state doesn't understand and doesn't trust her body.

PART 2

Reclaim Your Body

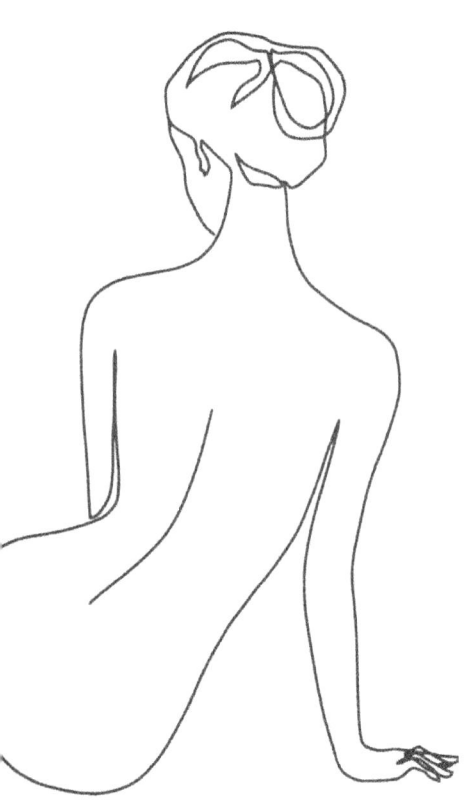

"Transform your relationship with your body and thrive in all aspects of your life."

IT'S TIME!

As women living in this time in history, we are presented with a unique opportunity to reclaim our identity, power, and natural mind-body-emotions connection.

We must restructure, rewire, and expand our understanding of and relationship with our bodies.

We must treat our bodies as allies instead of enemies.

In my work with my clients, this is a foundation for their results and success. Once they start learning and practicing it, they know how to listen to their bodies, workout for their unique situation, when to challenge themselves, and when to rest. Everything they do becomes more potent and effective in improving how they move and feel instead of contributing to their decline. The positive effects go beyond their physical body to reach every aspect of their lives!

"I suffered from back pain, neck pain, and headaches. My posture was poor and contributed to my aches and pains daily. My work with Rucsandra has noticeably eliminated pain. I can move with ease and have a sense of space in my body and my mind. I feel stronger, younger, healthier and happier." - **Robin Greer**

The women I work with start feeling stronger, more flexible, and more confident every year, not less. They reclaim their bodies *and their lives, and they do so with ease* and faster than they ever thought possible.

And so can YOU… *once you embrace your superpower and hone its power!*

Your body and life will never be the same once you know how to use it.

Are you ready?

A woman's superpower to unlock her natural body-mind-emotions connection, vitality, and confidence at any age is…

YOUR SUPERPOWER: AWARENESS

But it's not just any old kind of awareness. It's a refined, specific, subtle, and keen kind of Awareness. I'm excited to guide you in understanding this Awareness in a unique way that will give you unprecedented control of your body, mind, and emotions.

This is Capital A Awareness, and it will be referred to with Capital A throughout this book.

As a woman, you have the powerful ability to be aware of your physical, mental, and emotional states, which are all intertwined and experienced within your body.

This ability enables you to listen to your body and understand its messages. *It is the superpower that allows you to know and recognize your needs and respond to them accordingly.*

First and foremost, it's about being aware of your body *before understanding your mental and emotional states as they're expressed through it.*

To begin the process of "awakening" your Awareness, you must start with your physical body.

If your body feels tense or restricted, your ability to distinguish sensations is reduced and distorted.

Learning how to direct your attention, focus, and intention toward your body is crucial.

Once honed and developed, Awareness will transform your relationship with your body, dissolve the body-mind-emotions disconnect and *reveal your power to change the conditions in your body and your life*. It is the secret key to your health, vitality, and radiance.

> *"Your program has helped me change my relationship with my body, as well as my ability to breathe more deeply to nourish my body. I have a greater awareness and even the confidence that the balance in my body can be restored. I have a profound respect for your knowledge not only about the body but also of the mind."* - **Sylvia Korimsek.**

I have created a Practical Guide to help you awaken your superpower and reconnect your body, mind, and emotions.

The journey begins by connecting with your body, feeling, sensing, and becoming aware of it.

"To improve how you feel, you must first feel your body."

PRACTICE GUIDE FOR YOUR BODY

To cultivate Awareness, you need to focus on one specific area of your body and gradually expand your connection with it. Concentrating on one area and activity before extending the practice to another area and eventually to your entire body is essential.

To help you get started, let's focus on the movements of your ribcage during breathing. We take an average of about 22,000 breaths daily, and even the slightest correction in your breathing habits can profoundly improve how you feel.

This is what happens with your ribcage when you breathe correctly:

1. During the inhalation, your ribcage expands its volume vertically, horizontally, and from front to back.
2. During the exhalation, your ribcage contracts its volume vertically, horizontally, and from front to back.

However, due to tightness, stress, and injuries to the ribcage, shoulders, neck, or lower back, normal ribcage expansion and contraction may be restricted, affecting different parts of the body and leading to discomfort and tension throughout.

Proper breathing requires precise movements executed by the shoulders, spine, ribcage, and abdomen muscles. However, when certain body areas are tight or restricted, these movements become impeded, leading to discomfort, pain, and injuries.

Let's explore together the current patterns in your body when you inhale.

EXERCISE – BODY AWARENESS: BREATHING

We will focus on the inhalation here, and then you can expand the exercise to the exhalation.

How you inhale can have different effects on your body: it can increase tension and discomfort or have a tension-relief quality; therefore, it is not enough to only notice the depth of your inhalations.

Step 1 – Inhalation

You can perform this exercise in a seated position or while lying down. Focus all your attention on your breathing. Observe the sensations while you inhale: how it feels when you pull the air in through your nostrils, up through the nose, and down through your throat into your lungs.

Focus on each of the following questions for 3-4 inhales and note down your answers. Print out these pages and write your answers under each question.

1. Can you feel the two sides of your ribcage expanding?

   _____
   _____
   _____

2. How about the back of the ribcage?

   _____
   _____
   _____

3. Can you feel the front of the ribcage expanding? Is it more in the upper part, the lower part, or both?

   _____
   _____
   _____

4. Is your inhale expanding only your ribcage or your abdomen as well?

   _____
   _____
   _____

5. Can you feel only your abdomen expanding but not the ribcage?

_____
_____
_____

6. Is there any sensation in your shoulders or neck?

_____
_____
_____

7. Any sensation in the back of your head?

_____
_____
_____

8. Are your shoulders lifting?

_____
_____
_____

9. Is your neck tensing up?

_____
_____
_____

10. Can you tell if one side of your ribcage is expanding more than the other?

_____
_____
_____

11. Is your chest lifting and the back of your ribcage pulling forward, extending your thoracic spine?

_____
_____
_____

12. Is your inhale expanding the area between your shoulder blades?

_____
_____
_____

13. Can you feel your shoulder blades moving on your ribcage?

_____
_____
_____

14. Are you tensing up your jaw?

_____
_____
_____

15. Is your tongue on the floor of your mouth or pressing against the roof of your mouth?

___

16. Is your abdomen expanding and pulling your lumbar spine forward simultaneously?

___

17. What else can you feel during your inhale?

___

18. How do you feel emotionally as you keep your attention on your inhales?

___

19. Are you calm or getting restless, frustrated, or agitated?

___

Good! Now, take a moment to reflect on any insights you gained during this exercise and write them down.

Insights

If you stopped before completing all the questions or writing down your insights, that's okay.

Take a moment to acknowledge and celebrate the fact that you started. You can always return and gradually expand to more questions as your awareness grows.

Every question in the list above is important as your answers reveal the presence or absence of various patterns of movement and tension in your body.

When you are ready, proceed with…

Step 2 – Exhalation

Repeat the process for your exhale, focusing on different areas of your ribcage, abdomen, shoulders, and neck. Note down your insights.

Step 3 – Correct your breathing patterns

Once you become aware of your breathing patterns, you can use this knowledge to release tension, improve spinal movement, calm your nervous system, aid in injury healing, and create a deeper connection between your body and mind.

For example, if you notice that your inhales only expand the front of your ribcage, it means that your thoracic spine is not moving enough during your breathing. Each inhale creates more tension and restriction in your thoracic spine, which can affect your entire body. This can eventually lead to problems in your neck, shoulders, and lumbar spine.

To correct this breathing pattern, focus on expanding the back of your ribcage as much as you're expanding the front of your ribcage.

You take an average of 22,000 inhales every day. If each one *only* expands the front of your ribcage, it is crucial to change your breathing habits first. Otherwise, other methods to alleviate neck, shoulder, or lower back pain will only have a limited effect.

If your inhalations cause your abdomen to expand but not your ribcage, it indicates that the joints in your ribcage, spine, and shoulders are not benefiting from the natural movements of effective inhalation. This increases tightness, restriction, and limited movement in those joints.

To correct this breathing pattern, begin to expand the rib cage during inhalation to improve your ribcage, shoulder, and spine movements.

Understanding the patterns of tension and habits in your body is the most essential step towards achieving greater ease and freedom of movement.

It is a powerful practice, and it will take time to feel all areas of your ribcage in relation to the rest of your body during both your inhalation and exhalation. As you continue to practice, you will become more mindful of the movement of your ribcage in relation to the rest of your body, leading to improved breathing habits.

It is a practice

worth your time and effort

because each breath will then

help you release tension and discomfort

rather than contribute

to the patterns that created them.

This practice also serves as a form of meditation that can improve your mental and emotional well-being and allow you to connect with yourself on a level you might not have thought possible.

Concentrate on your body for the next four weeks by learning to perceive new sensations and enhancing your Awareness of different areas of your body.

Step 4 - Start a Victories Book

Remember to celebrate every new insight, realization, and even the slightest increase in your Awareness.

As part of my programs and courses, I always recommend that my clients maintain a dedicated notebook for documenting their physical improvements, accomplishments, breakthroughs, and successes—a Victories Book—no matter how small or big they are.
This notebook is an incredibly valuable tool that proves its worth during times of discouragement. By reviewing their notes in the pages of this notebook, they can effortlessly shift the balance of their thoughts and mental state.

In this process, they expand their capacity to:

- Notice when they feel good, when their body is relaxed, and when an area of their body has significantly improved
- Understand their body's more subtle messages
- Correctly interpret their body's signals

- Accurately distinguish between various sensations like soreness, ache, tenderness, and discomfort
- Pay attention to their breathing
- Know if they feel tension caused by emotional strain, stress, or physical tightness.
- Be aware of how different mental and emotional states affect their body.

Step 4 in the Breathing Awareness Exercise is the beginning of your own Victories Book. Now, buy yourself a new notebook with a beautiful cover that pleases you and begin recording your successes.

As you progress on your Awareness journey, the next step is understanding your thoughts and establishing a clear and effective connection between your mind and body. Follow the steps outlined in Part 2 of the Practice Guide.

"To use your mind to improve how you feel, you must first become aware of your thoughts."

PRACTICE GUIDE FOR YOUR MIND

In this section, you will explore how your thoughts impact your body. We'll start again in the body. Let's focus on an area of your body where you feel discomfort, tension, or tightness.

EXERCISE – THOUGHT AWARENESS

Please choose the area you want to concentrate on and write it below.

Area of the body

_____

_____

_____

_____

Step 1 – Physical sensations

Take note of your physical sensations first and write them down in a notebook or on these pages.

Bring your attention, focus, and awareness to the chosen area in your body. Please pay attention to every physical sensation you feel in that area and describe them in as much detail as possible. Observe which sensations are intense and which are not. Take note of the sharp, vivid sensations and the subtle ones that you can barely feel.

That is okay if you cannot initially feel anything beyond discomfort. Take a few minutes to focus on your breath and the sensations it generates. If you have already completed the Breathing Awareness exercise in Part 1 of the Practice Guide, you will be familiar with paying attention to your ribcage, neck, shoulders, and abdomen.

Write down the sensations you feel during breathing to serve as a guide.

Then, redirect your focus to the specific area of your body you wish to connect with. Observe it with the same level of attention you give to your ribcage during breathing and notice additional sensations. If required, you may repeat the Breathing Awareness Exercise.

Next, we will explore how your thoughts affect the physical sensations in your body.

Step 2 – Thoughts

Start by writing down anything that comes to mind as you focus on the area where you feel discomfort. Here are a few examples to get you going:

> I'm tired of the pain/discomfort/tightness in this area.
> It's getting worse.
> It felt a little better after the last session of _____, but it didn't last.
> I don't know what to do; nothing is working.
> I'm so frustrated.
> Something must be wrong.
> I might be feeling less discomfort today.

Use the lined page below to write down everything that comes to mind without censoring. Set a timer for 20 minutes and keep writing. If you notice specific thoughts are repeated, keep writing. Bring everything out of your mind and onto the paper.

Do your thoughts revolve mainly around what's not working, or are you also considering progress and improvement? Write down your insights.

Insights

_____
_____
_____
_____
_____
_____
_____
_____
_____
_____
_____
_____

Focusing on what you don't want and everything going wrong is easy when you're uncomfortable or in pain. Your mind gets used to seeing difficulties and obstacles and focusing on discomfort and pain.

Awareness means recognizing and understanding your thoughts relating to your physical sensations. It also means paying attention to what is going right, to everything you are already doing well, and to every improvement, no matter how small.

When you shift your focus from what's not working to what is, the tension in your body will ease, reducing discomfort.

Step 3 – Shifting the focus

Now, you will write down things that are going well in your body. Set a timer for 20 minutes and continue writing until it goes off.

If you find this challenging and want to stop, that is okay. Acknowledge what you feel, take a breath, and do it anyway or return to it later. Keep looking for things to write down. Be gentle and take it easy on yourself. Give yourself the freedom to explore this process with curiosity and self-directed kindness.

If you have trouble coming up with something, remember that after completing Part 1 of the Practice Guide, your Awareness of your ribcage during inhalation is sharper and more refined. Write a detailed list of how your Awareness has improved.

Now, focus again on the area where tension and discomfort were present and notice any new sensations. Write down your insights.

Insights:

_____
_____
_____
_____
_____
_____
_____
_____
_____
_____

Step 4 – Update your Victories Book

Record your insights and realizations in your Victories Book.

To help my clients increase their physical and mental Awareness, I have developed a process called Health Essentials. During these sessions, I help my clients recognize and become aware of patterns of resistance and restriction in their bodies and minds and teach them how to overcome them.

At the end of each Health Essentials session, the participants share their insights, realizations, and a-ha moments. Their heightened Awareness is anchored in their bodies and minds through sharing and witnessing. They develop a deeper, more precise, and more powerful understanding of their bodies and minds.

Every time you record a new insight, a-ha moment, or realization in your Victories Book, you anchor it into your body and mind; you make it your new reality.

"To improve how you feel, you must feel your emotions."

PRACTICE GUIDE FOR YOUR EMOTIONS

This section will focus on how your emotions affect your body.

If you experience any resistance to the exercise below and want to close this book, that is okay.

Acknowledge what you feel, take a breath, and do it anyway or return to it later. This is a deep exploration, and it requires time. Be gentle with yourself and proceed at your own pace. Give yourself the freedom to explore this process with curiosity and self-directed kindness.

EXERCISE – EMOTION AWARENESS

We will concentrate on an unpleasant emotion that has been with you for a long time or is more recent.

Identify the emotion you want to focus on and write it below. It can be sadness, anger, worry, fear, shame, guilt.

Emotion

_____

_____

_____

Step 1 - Physical sensations

Notice where in your body you feel this emotion. What physical sensations are you experiencing? Do you feel any tightness, constriction, tension, or contraction? Take note of your breathing as you focus on this emotion.

Please pay attention to every physical sensation related to this emotion and describe them in as much detail as possible. Observe which sensations are intense and which are not. Note any sharp, vivid, or subtle sensations.

Give your emotion a voice. Write down the physical manifestation of this emotion in a notebook or print the lined page below.

Set a timer for 20 minutes and continue writing until it goes off. Use extra paper if you need it. Keep writing.

If you find that the intensity of your emotion increases when you focus on it, stay with it. Try shaking your arms, standing up and pacing around the room, taking a few deep breaths, and then returning to your writing.

Good, take a moment to acknowledge and celebrate yourself for writing everything down!

Next, we will return to your breathing awareness exercise.

Step 2 – Breathing Awareness

Set a timer for 5 minutes and focus on your breath. You can use the questions in the Breathing Awareness Exercise as a guide or self-direct your attention to different areas of your ribcage.

Keep your attention on your inhales and exhales. If your mind wanders, bring it back to your breath. If it wanders again, bring it back without becoming frustrated. Be patient, kind, and compassionate toward yourself. Your mind will wander, and staying calm and aware of it is part of the practice.

When your timer goes off, reconnect with your emotion and notice its intensity after focusing on your breath for only 5 minutes. If it's still intense, set your timer again and repeat. Then, write down your insights.

Insights:

_____
_____
_____
_____
_____
_____
_____

_____

_____

_____

Step 3 – Release the emotion in your body

With your attention connected to your body through your breath, it is time to use your Awareness to soften, loosen, and release the emotion.

Set your timer for 10 minutes and focus on your breathing again. Now, imagine that you can send your breath precisely in the area in your body where you felt your emotion in Step 1 of this exercise.

Imagine your inhales reaching your neck, solar plexus, shoulder, hip, and lower back, wherever you identify your emotion. At this stage of your practice, you might think, "There are no lungs in my hips or lower back. How can I send my breath there?"

Indeed, there are no lungs in any area of your body except in your ribcage. But, with an increased Awareness of how your ribcage expands during inhalation, you can extend the sensation of expansion anywhere in your body.

Use your mind and imagination, and when the picture of your hips or lower back expanding on your inhalation is formed and strengthened, you will become aware of the physical sensation of this expansion. If you find this more challenging, that is okay. Practice for a few minutes and return to this part of the exercise later. *Most importantly, be kind and patient with yourself. You are learning a new way to connect your body, mind, and emotions.*

When your timer goes off, feel your emotion, feel its level, and write down your insights.

Insights:

_____
_____
_____
_____
_____
_____
_____
_____

Step 4 – Update your Victories Book

Record your successes in your Victories Book during the next few days and weeks.

As you practice the exercises in this book, you will gradually experience a profound transformation in your life. You will notice that your body has less tension and discomfort, and you will have an increased ability to remain calm during stressful situations. You will learn to apply body-mind-emotions Awareness in your daily life, helping you navigate every situation with ease and inner power.

Here are some of my clients' victories to inspire and encourage you to notice and celebrate your own:

> *"Going to the dentist has always caused me enormous fear, which created great tension in my body. But yesterday, everything was different. I practiced what I learned in your program. I used my breathing and connection with my body to prepare myself and enter a calm state before arriving at my dentist's office. And I was able to maintain this calm state throughout the whole time. This is truly empowering!"*

> *"I'm having a weekend with such ease, including (remarkably) a cable transition to a new plan and equipment! In the past, doing that kind of thing (especially new plan negotiations) put me in a frustrating spin, but not today! So much has turned from ouch to ease."*

"They are replacing computers at my office, and the process is far from progressing smoothly. This would have been highly stressful and upsetting for me in the past, but not anymore. Everything and everyone around me is in complete chaos, but I am calm, centered, and in control of my mind and emotions."

FINAL THOUGHTS

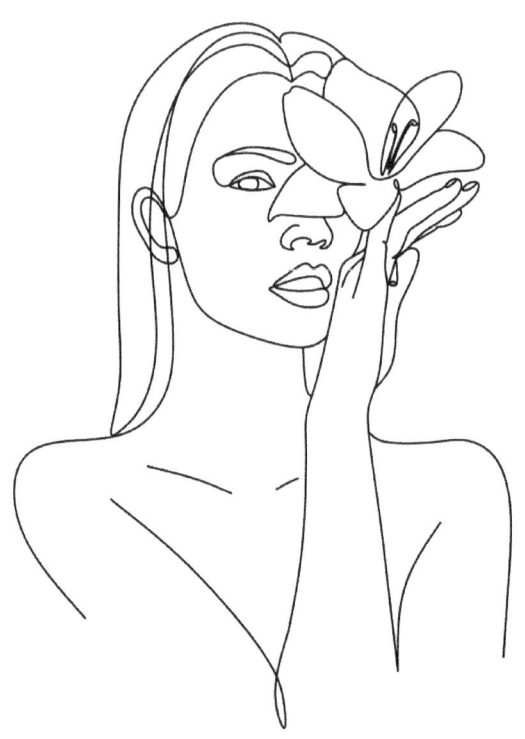

INDESTRUCTIBLE CONFIDENCE

Improving your breathing awareness is a first step. As you progress, you can expand your attention to different body parts, such as your feet, ankles, knees, hips, neck, shoulders, and lower back. By doing this, you will also understand how these different body parts relate.

This understanding will allow you to avoid injuries, engage in the appropriate form of exercise for your situation, improve your physical, mental, and emotional well-being, and benefit more profoundly from any relaxation technique, stress-release practice, or meditation session.

Improving your awareness of your body and its movements will help you better understand yourself and achieve higher self-awareness.

As you continue practicing and internalizing this awareness, you will take ownership of your body and well-being. You will not be susceptible to external factors influenced by the latest discussion on social media or societal expectations that aging inevitably leads to pain and restricted movement.

You will learn to trust your body.

So, what does this mean for your health and well-being?

In practical and immediate terms, what this really means is that you will be able to:

1. Eliminate discomfort, tension, restrictions, tightness, and movement limitations with less effort and time than you thought possible.
2. Improve your strength, flexibility, mobility, and agility as you age instead of settling for the idea that your body is falling apart just because you're getting older.
3. Enter deep states of relaxation that are profoundly healing.

With consistent practice, the benefits will gradually expand to include an increased awareness of your thoughts and emotions. You will know *in your body* if they increase tension and discomfort or help you release them.

In other words, you will become aware of *the physical manifestations of thoughts and emotions before they become injuries or chronic conditions*. You will notice subtle shifts in your body when you think specific thoughts and experience certain emotions before they manifest as relentless tension, discomfort, or pain. You can then deliberately choose your thoughts and be present with your emotions to help your body feel better.

You will begin to feel and know—in your body and without a doubt—when to challenge your body, when to take it gently or rest, exactly how much and when to sleep, and what foods to eat.

You will learn to trust your intuition. You will come to understand that just as nature has seasons, so has your body, and so have you. You will adjust your self-care routine to align with your body's needs.

Ultimately, Awareness will forever change the way you:

- Feel your body
- Understand your body
- Relate to your body
- Connect with your body
- Move your body
- Listen to your body
- Heal your body
- Live in your body

Awareness will become an integral part of your life.

You will gain an outstanding understanding of your body and yourself.

You will begin to trust yourself and your body's capacity to improve, restore, and heal at any age.

You will achieve a level of self-confidence that was previously unimaginable.

> "Before I met you, my life was often filled with physical and emotional pain, from frozen shoulders to feeling emotionally vulnerable like a little fish swimming upstream. Today, I feel in control of my body, mind, and emotions. You have taught me to listen to my body and have given me countless tools to deal with life's challenges. I am no longer running from one practitioner to another, hoping that they will be able to end the pain in my body. Instead, I am attending your program when I need a soothing voice and guidance on how to move my body and rest if that is needed. Stress has left my vocabulary, thanks to you and your teachings. Every day, I find a way to include a live or recorded class, knowing that at the end, I will feel so relaxed and at ease. I am grateful to be part of a wonderful community of people who, like me, are aging wonderfully. With much gratitude, Patricia"- **Patricia Poyntz**

WHAT'S NEXT?

In this book, we've discussed the historical obstacles to a woman's natural state of body-mind-emotions Awareness and connection.

Additionally, we have explored how being disconnected negatively affects a woman's body and life.

Then, we've discussed the life-changing benefits of transitioning from a disconnected state into a state of Awareness.

We practiced bringing your attention and focusing on your inhales, and I have given you the steps to increase your awareness of how your inhales affect your body.

We then expanded the practice to your thoughts and emotions.

I have also shared some remarkable successes achieved by women like yourself.

Now it's your time to step out of the disconnected state and into Awareness!

Begin with your breathing using the practice guide I provided. This is the first step in the process.

Gradually extend your practice until you establish a strong and clear connection with your entire body.

In this state of Awareness, you can observe and listen to your body's signals with unprecedented understanding, kindness, and compassion.

Imagine connecting with any area of your body experiencing discomfort and pain and easily discern if the discomfort is generated by stress or emotional strain or has a physical cause.

Imagine knowing exactly what to do to release tension and eliminate discomfort.

Imagine breaking free from the conditioning that has created the disconnected state.

Imagine reclaiming your power to transform how you feel physically, mentally, and emotionally.

This power is at your fingertips, and it starts with your body.

As we end this book, I encourage you to continue your journey towards Awareness. I have created a video training to guide you through the Inhalation Awareness Exercise, as explained in this book. I have also prepared a bonus video to lead you through the Exhalation Awareness Exercise. You can access this training for free by scanning the QR code below.

With love,

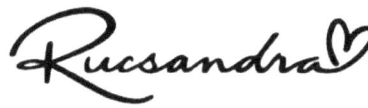

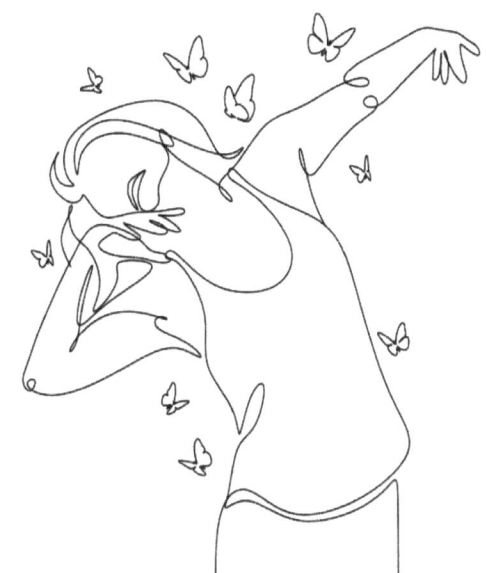

References

1. Hunter, C. W., Deer, T. R., Jones, M. R., Chien, G. C. C., D'Souza, R. S., Davis, T., Eldon, E. R., Esposito, M. F., Goree, J. H., Hewan-Lowe, L., Maloney, J. A., Mazzola, A. J., Michels, J. S., Layno-Moses, A., Patel, S., Tari, J., Weisbein, J. S., Goulding, K. A., Chhabra, A., & Hassebrock, J. (2022). Consensus Guidelines on Interventional Therapies for Knee Pain (STEP Guidelines) from the American Society of Pain and Neuroscience. *Journal of Pain Research*, 15, 2683–2745. https://doi.org/10.2147/JPR.S370469

2. Canada, H. (2019, August 8). *Canadian Pain Task Force Report: June 2019*. Www.canada.ca. https://www.canada.ca/en/health-canada/corporate/about-health-canada/public-engagement/external-advisory-bodies/canadian-pain-task-force/report-2019.html#intro

3. *Arthritis and Joint Pain | National Poll on Healthy Aging*. (n.d.). Www.healthyagingpoll.org. https://www.healthyagingpoll.org/reports-more/report/arthritis-and-joint-pain

4. Jonas, W. 2018 Women and Pain: Taking Control and Finding Relief https://healingworksfoundation.org/wp-content/uploads/2018/05/WomenandPain-White-Paper_051518_FNL_web.pdf

5. *Here's Why Women Are More Likely to Have Chronic* Pain. (n.d.). Cleveland Clinic. Retrieved May 6, 2024, from https://health.clevelandclinic.org/women-are-more-likely-to-have-chronic-pain-heres-why

6. *Pain or discomfort that prevents* activities. (2010, January 11). Statcan.gc.ca. https://www150.statcan.gc.ca/n1/pub/82-229-x/2009001/status/pdl-eng.htm

www.ingramcontent.com/pod-product-compliance
Lightning Source LLC
Chambersburg PA
CBHW040223040426
42333CB00051B/3425